TIMBI talks about ADDICTION

Helping Children Cope with a Parent's Addiction

by

Trish Healy Luna & Janet Healy Hellier

illustrated by

Mackenzie Mitchell

designed by

Lynette Sesler

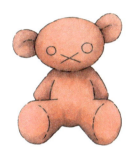

For Nick & Sami
With Everlasting Love,

Momma & Aunt Janet ♡

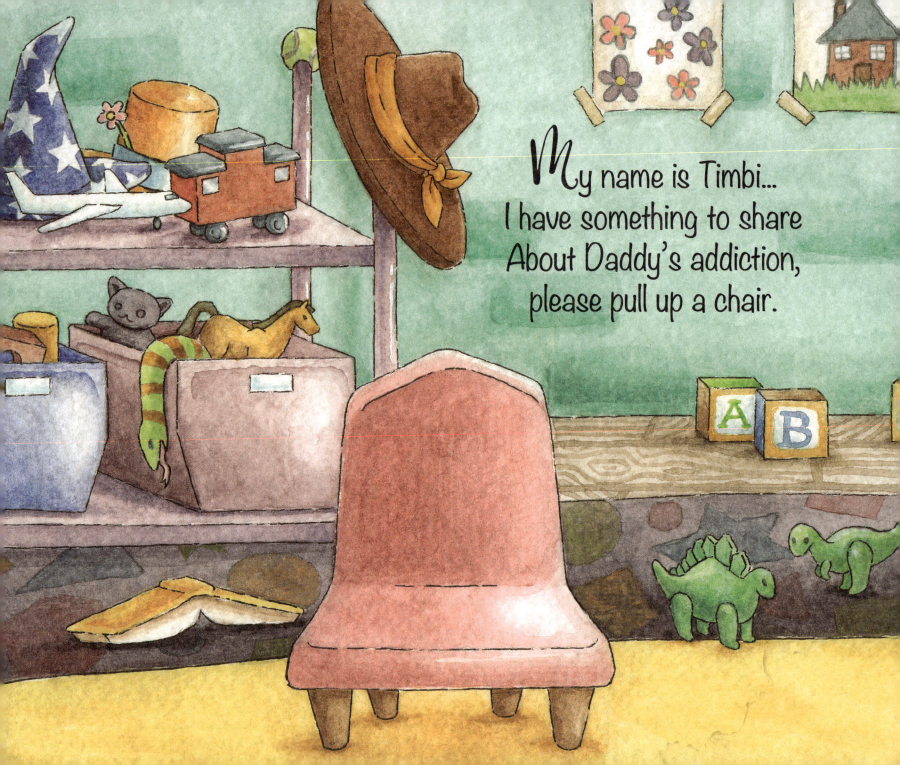

My name is Timbi...
I have something to share
About Daddy's addiction,
please pull up a chair.

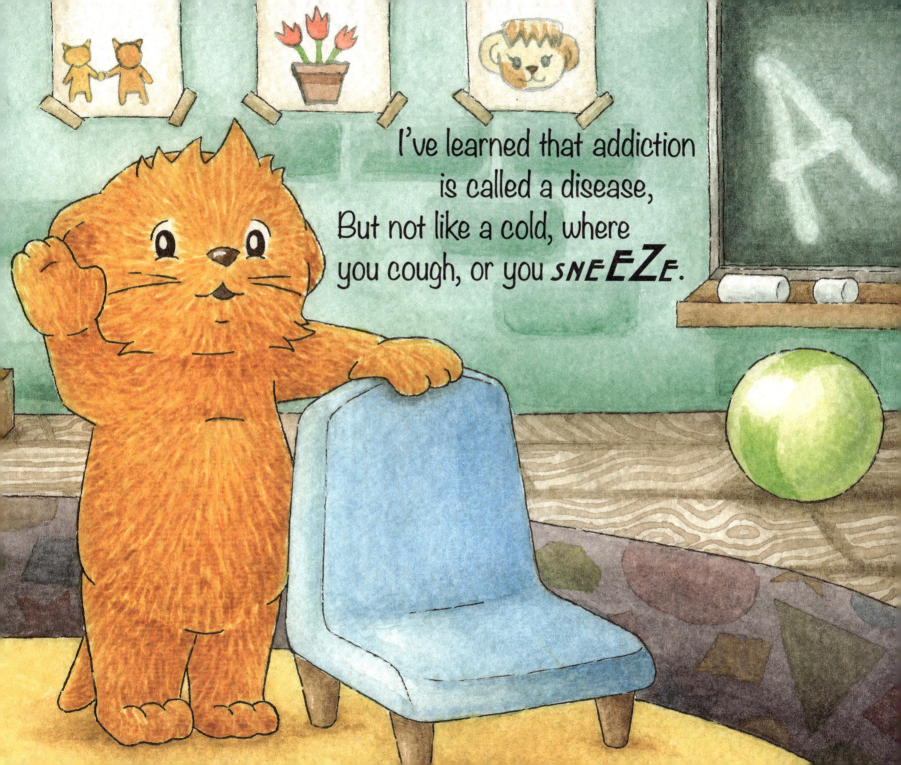

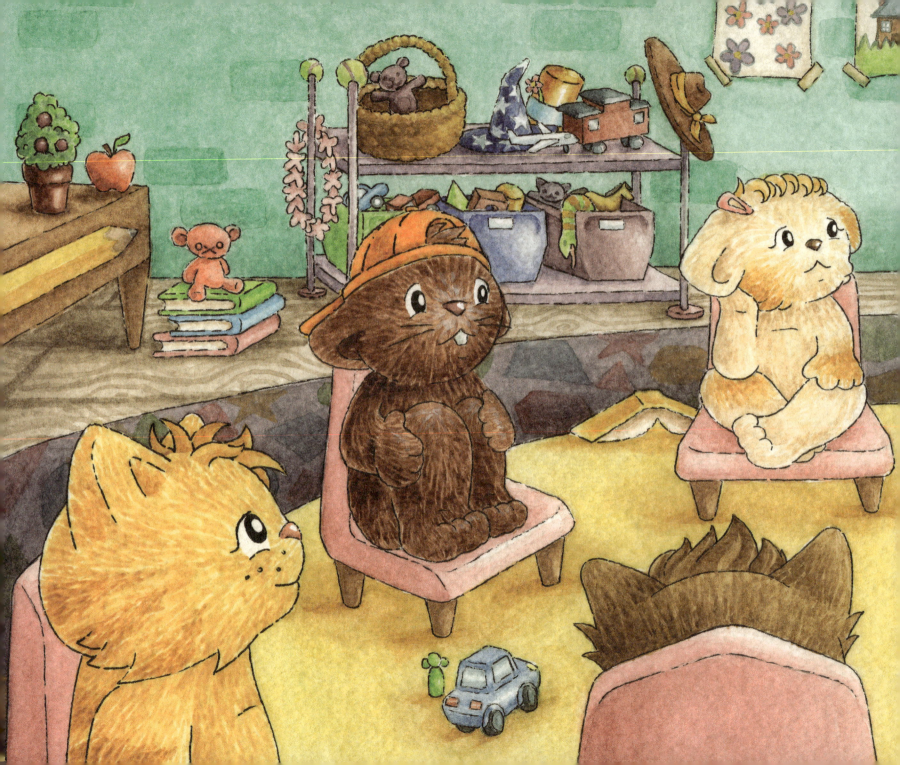

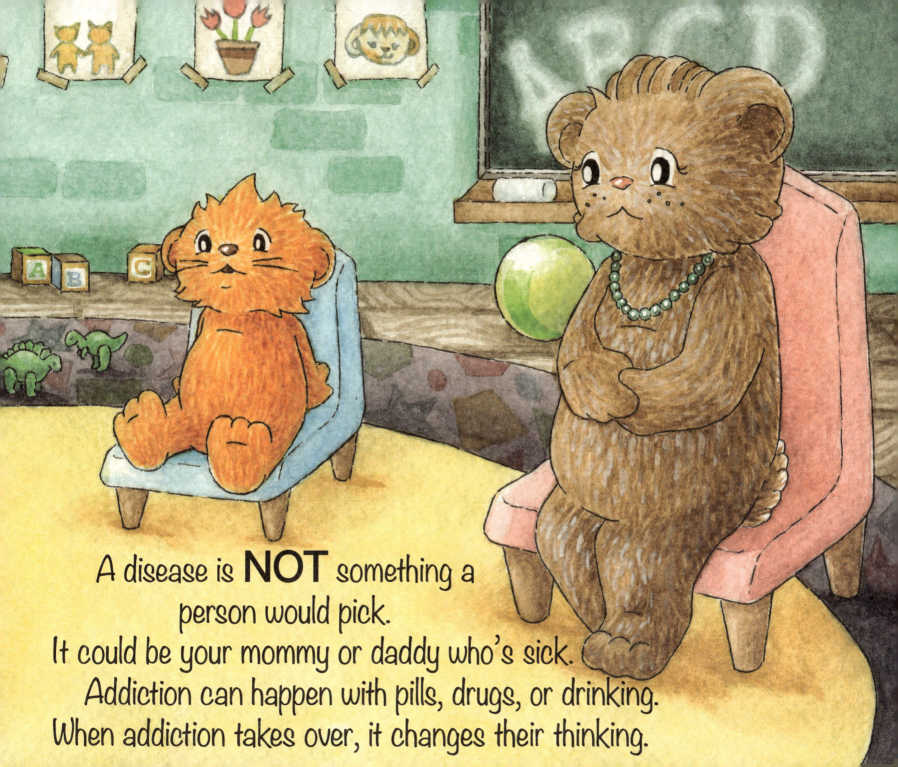

A disease is **NOT** something a person would pick.
It could be your mommy or daddy who's sick.
Addiction can happen with pills, drugs, or drinking.
When addiction takes over, it changes their thinking.

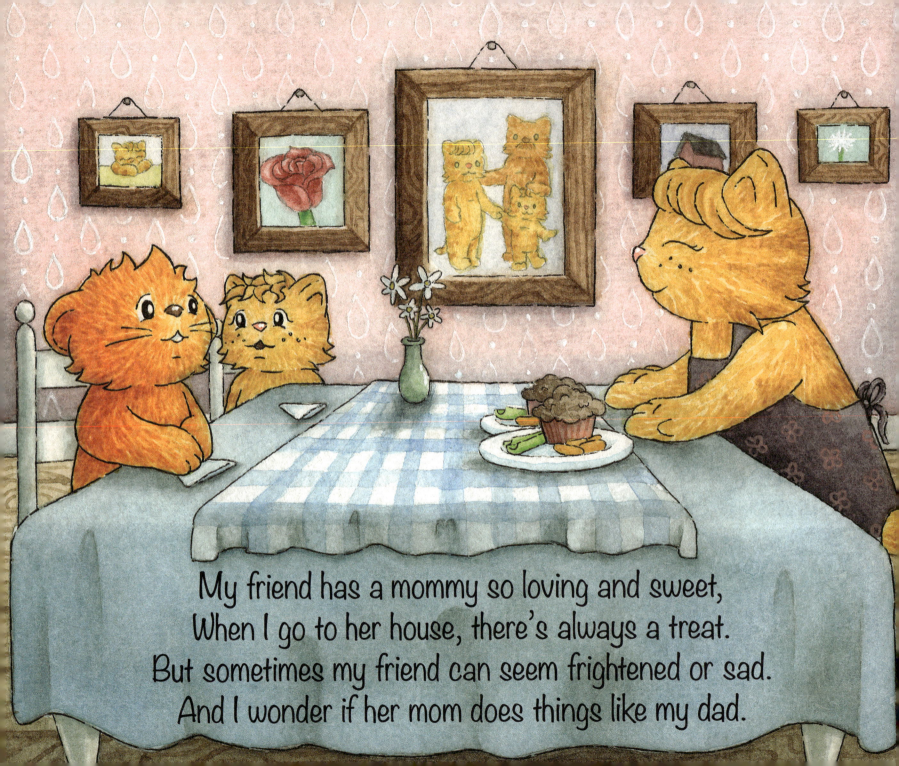

My friend has a mommy so loving and sweet,
When I go to her house, there's always a treat.
But sometimes my friend can seem frightened or sad.
And I wonder if her mom does things like my dad.

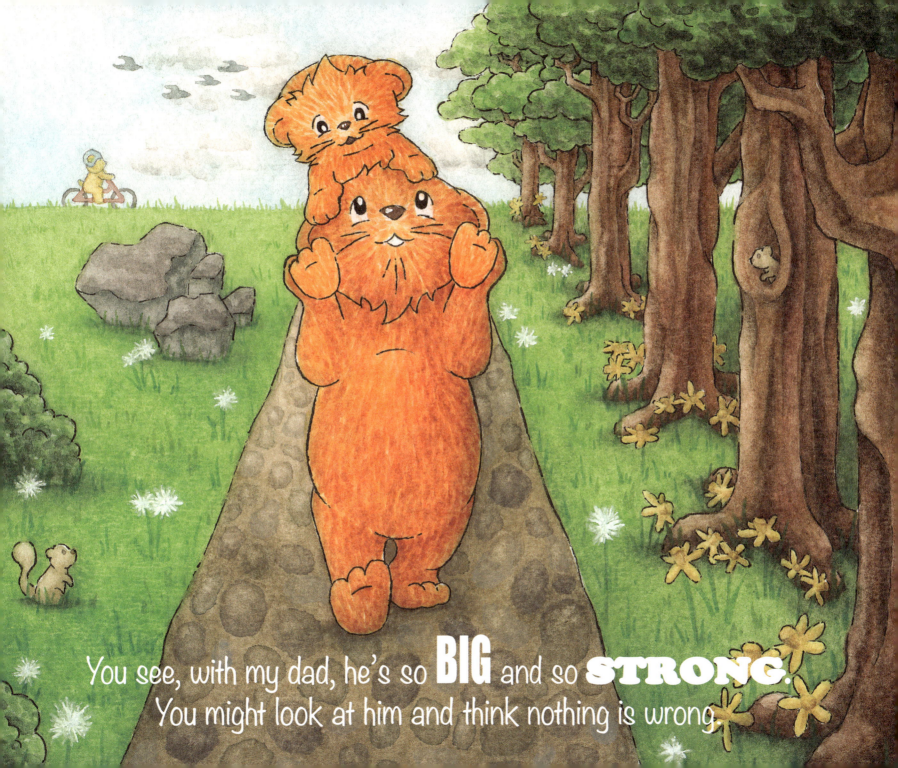

You see, with my dad, he's so **BIG** and so **STRONG**.
You might look at him and think nothing is wrong.

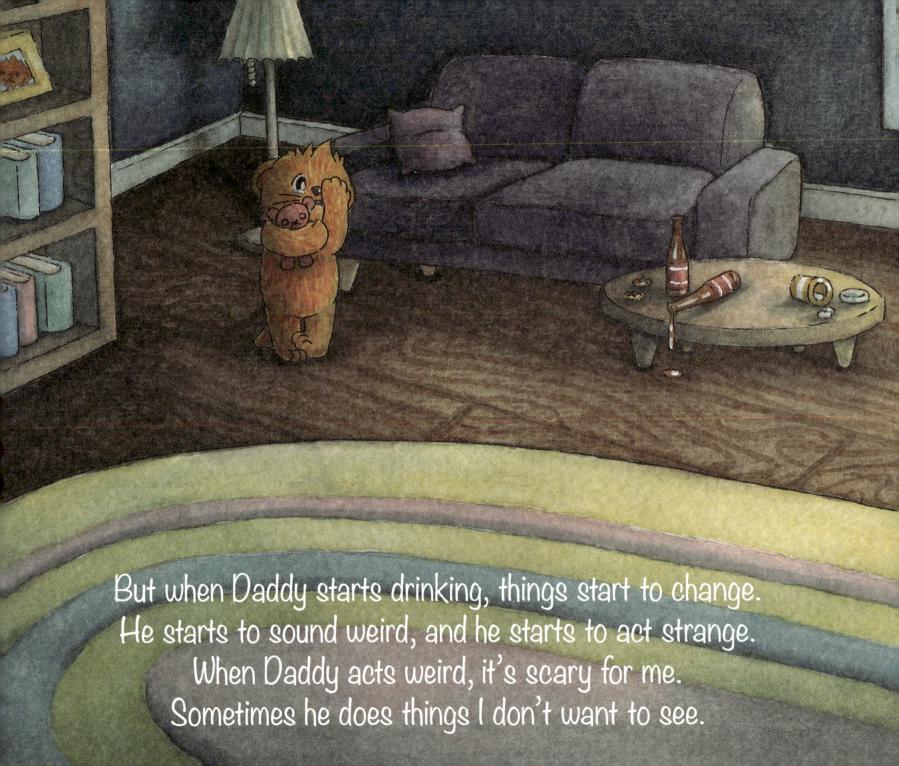

But when Daddy starts drinking, things start to change.
He starts to sound weird, and he starts to act strange.
When Daddy acts weird, it's scary for me.
Sometimes he does things I don't want to see.

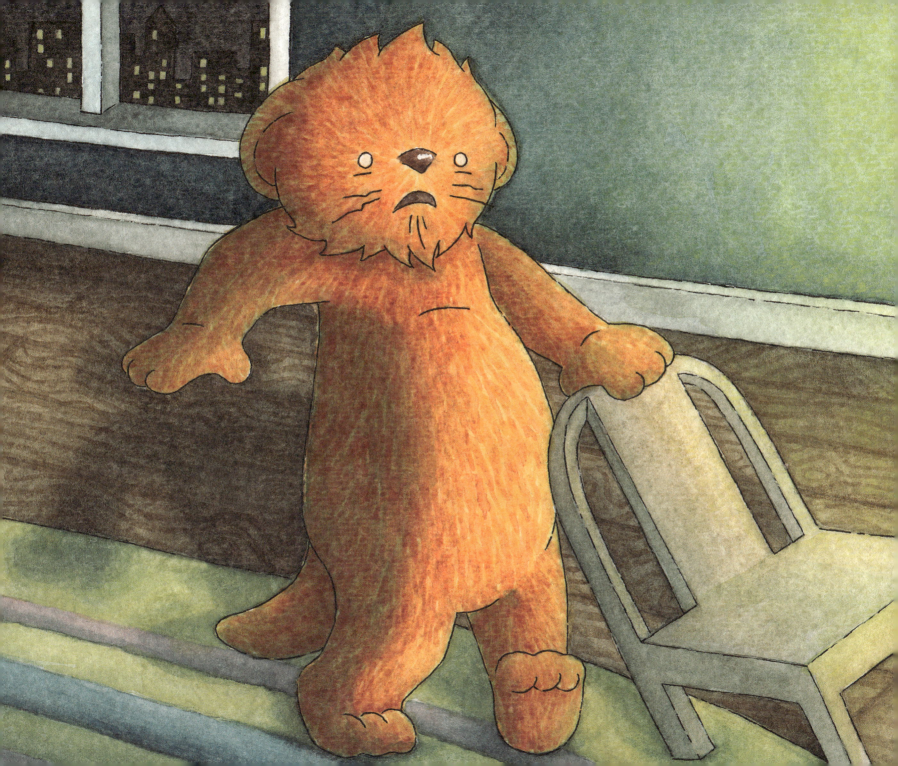

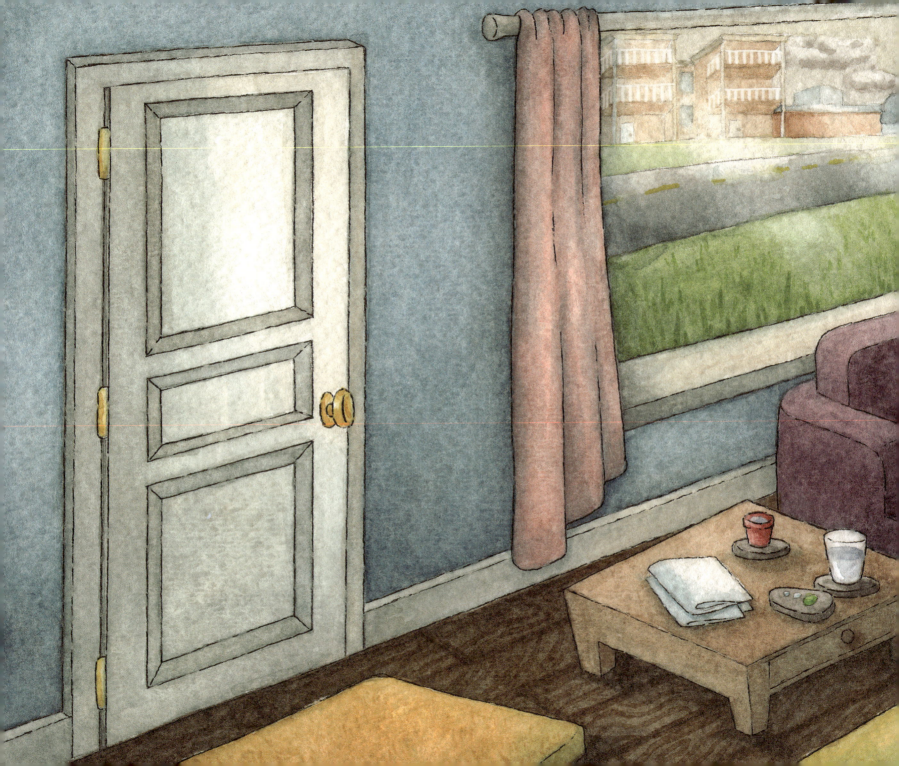

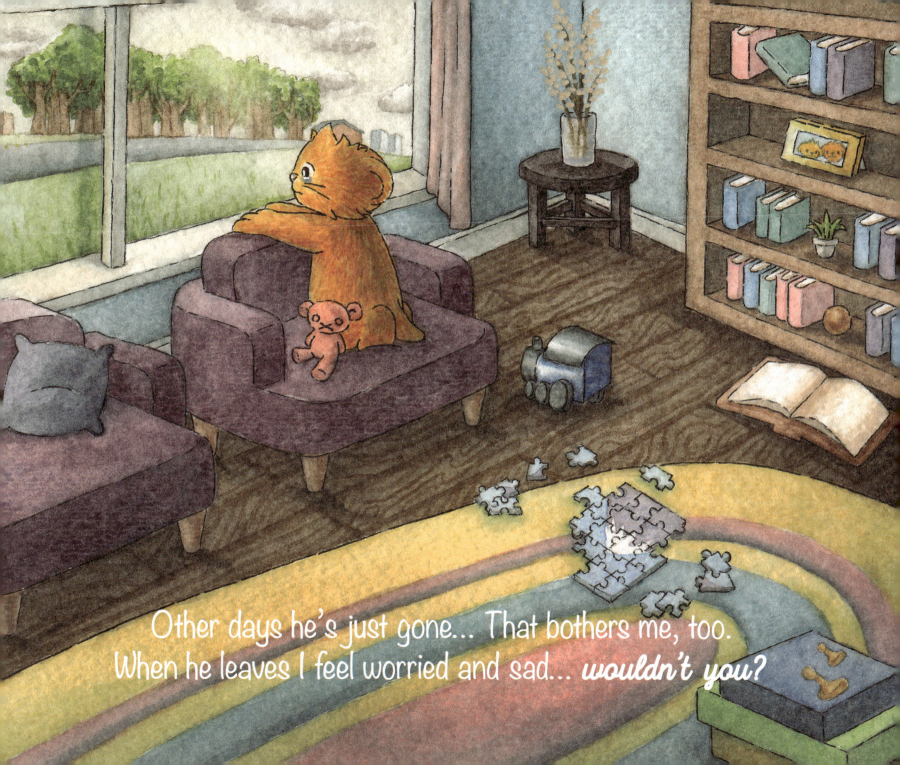

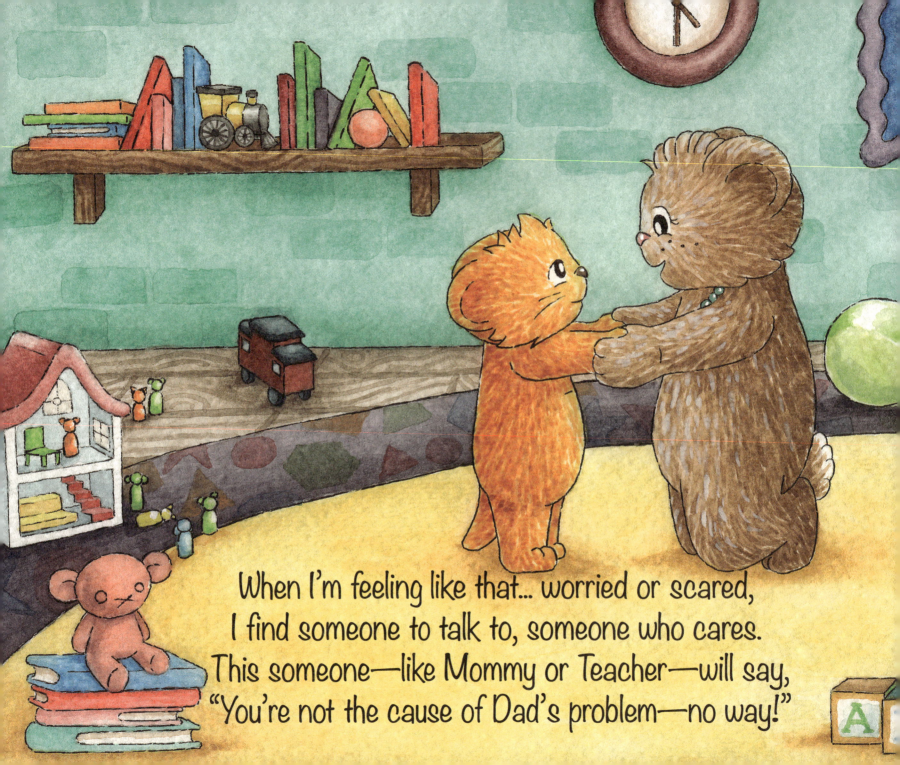

When I'm feeling like that... worried or scared,
I find someone to talk to, someone who cares.
This someone—like Mommy or Teacher—will say,
"You're not the cause of Dad's problem—no way!"

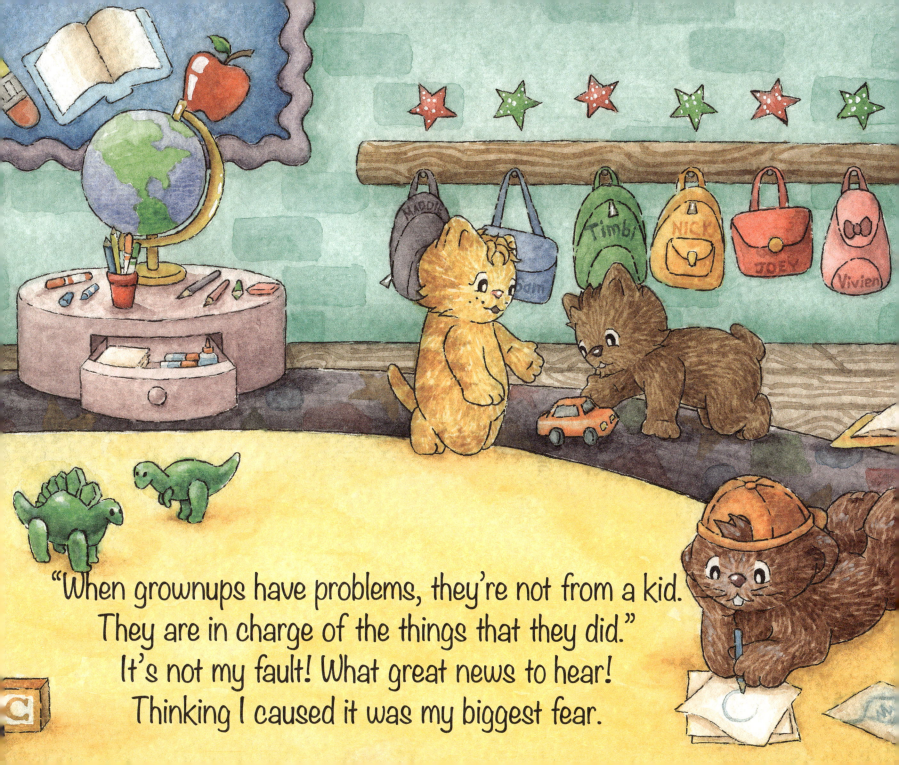

"When grownups have problems, they're not from a kid.
They are in charge of the things that they did."
It's not my fault! What great news to hear!
Thinking I caused it was my biggest fear.

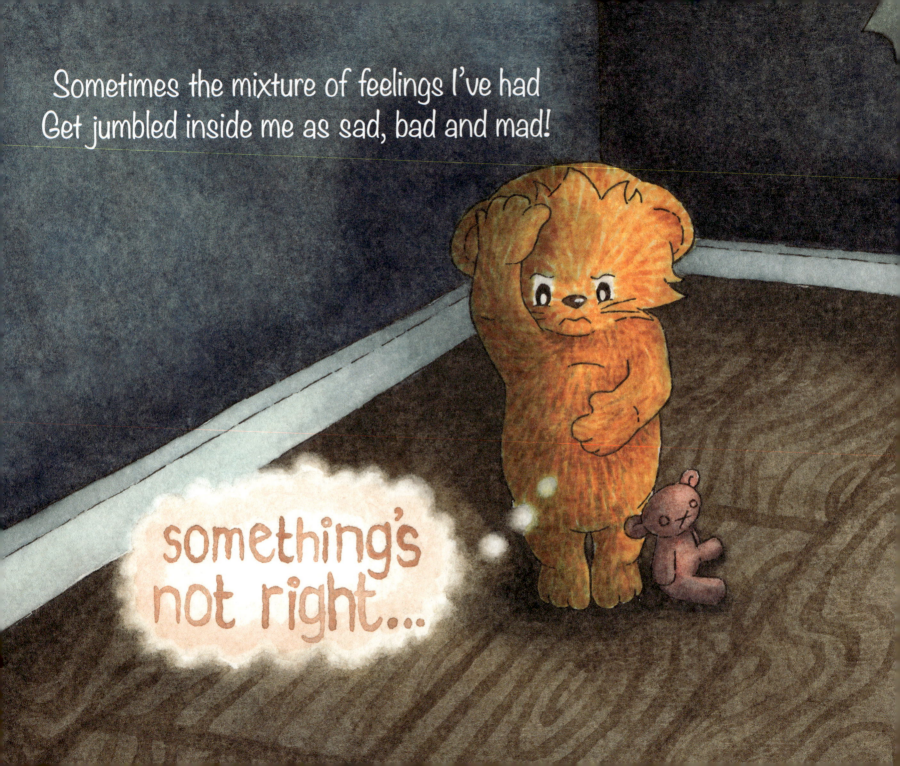

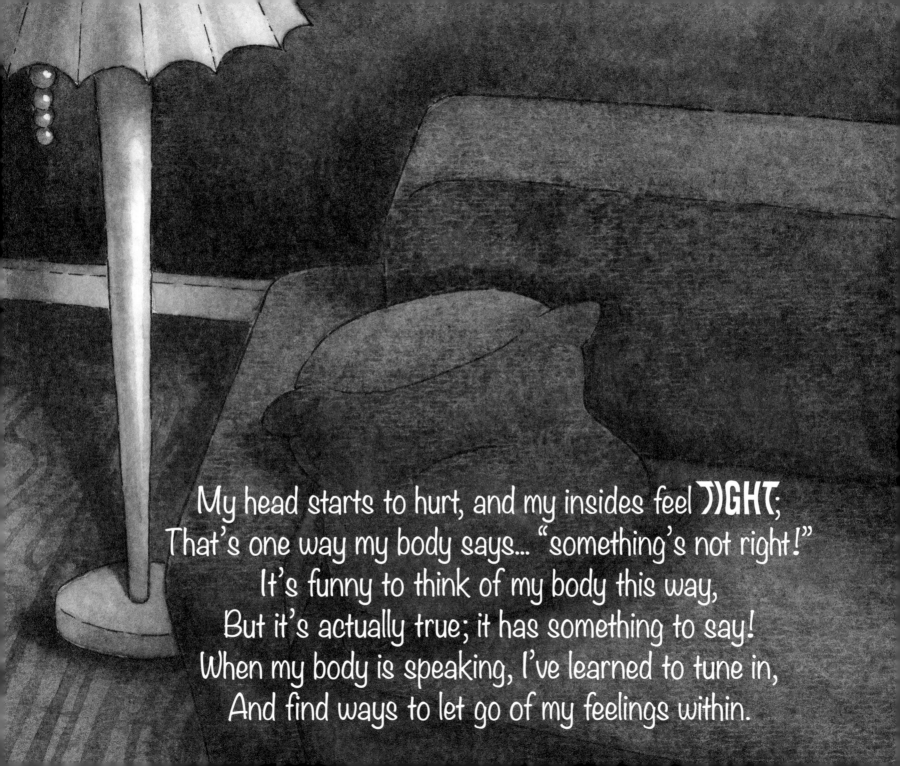

My head starts to hurt, and my insides feel TIGHT;
That's one way my body says... "something's not right!"
It's funny to think of my body this way,
But it's actually true; it has something to say!
When my body is speaking, I've learned to tune in,
And find ways to let go of my feelings within.

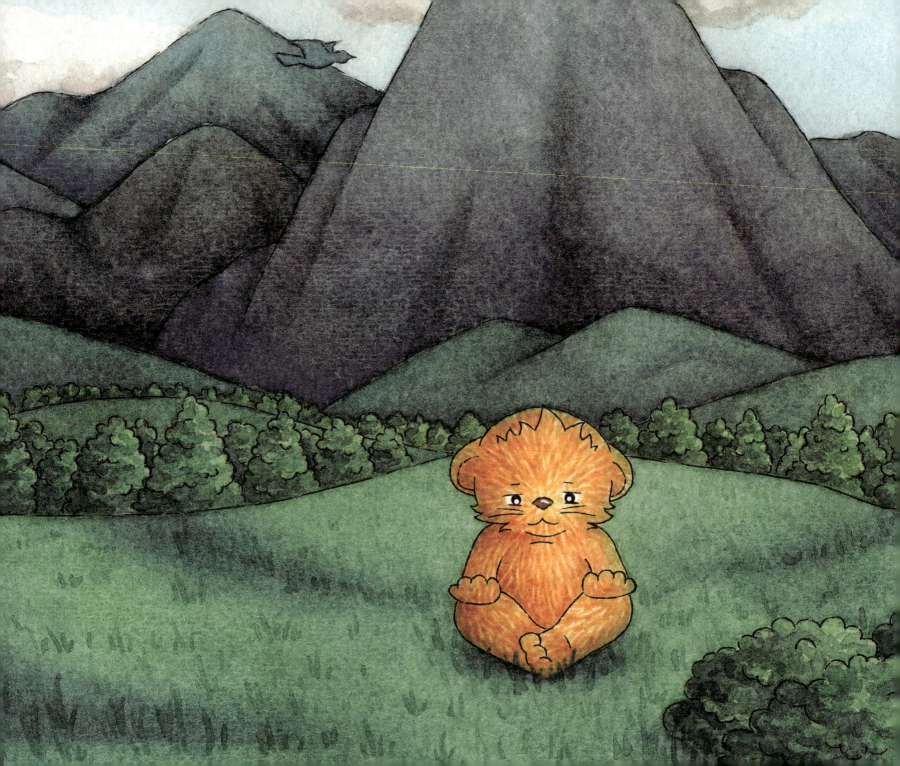

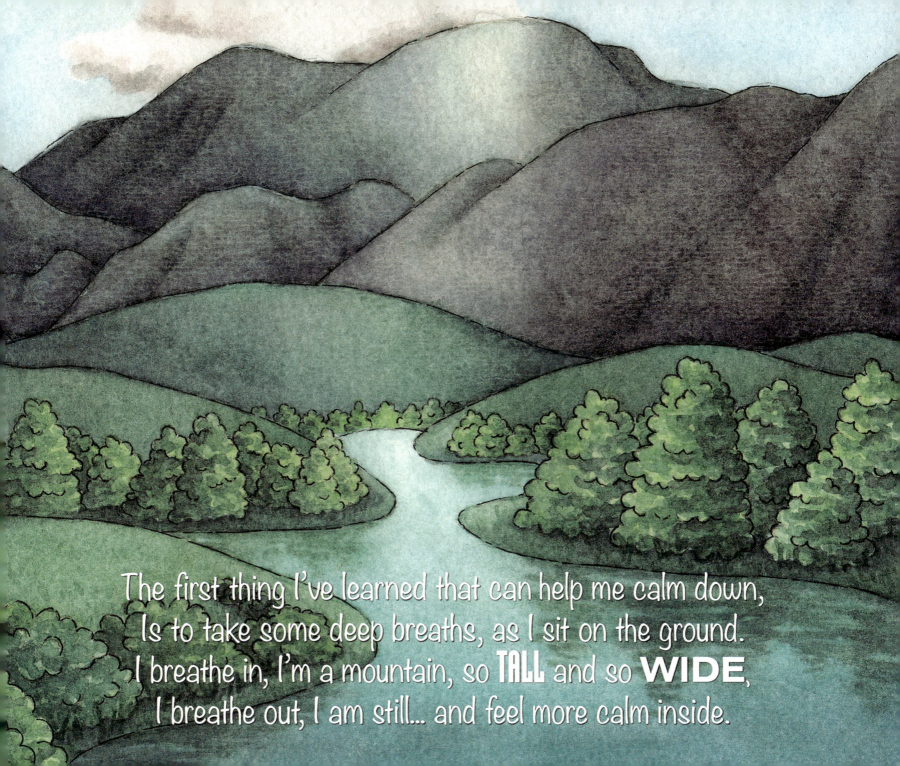

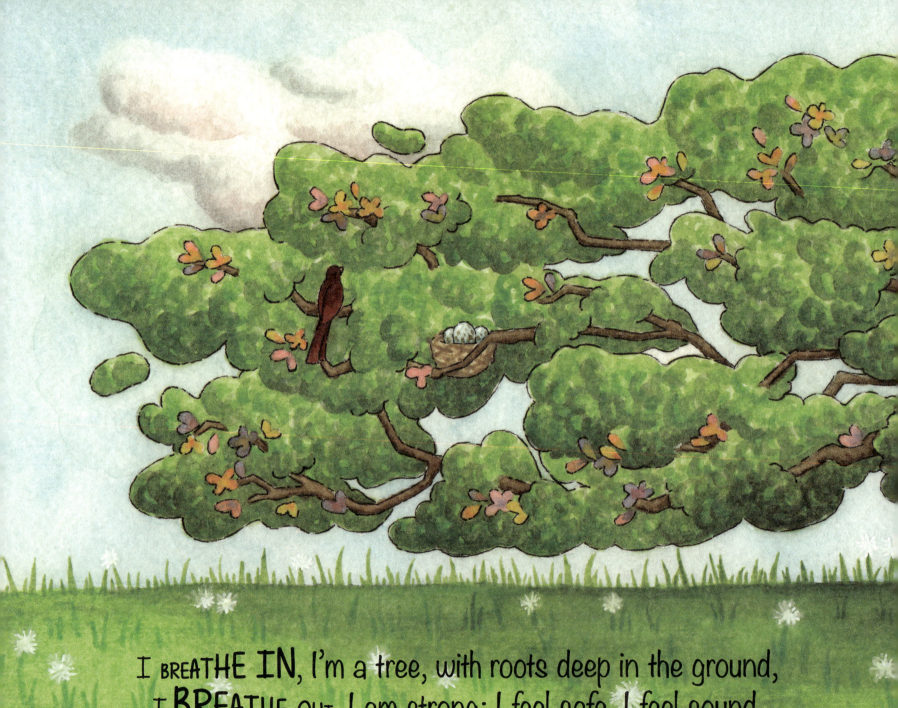

I BREATHE IN, I'm a tree, with roots deep in the ground,
I BREATHE OUT, I am strong; I feel safe, I feel sound.

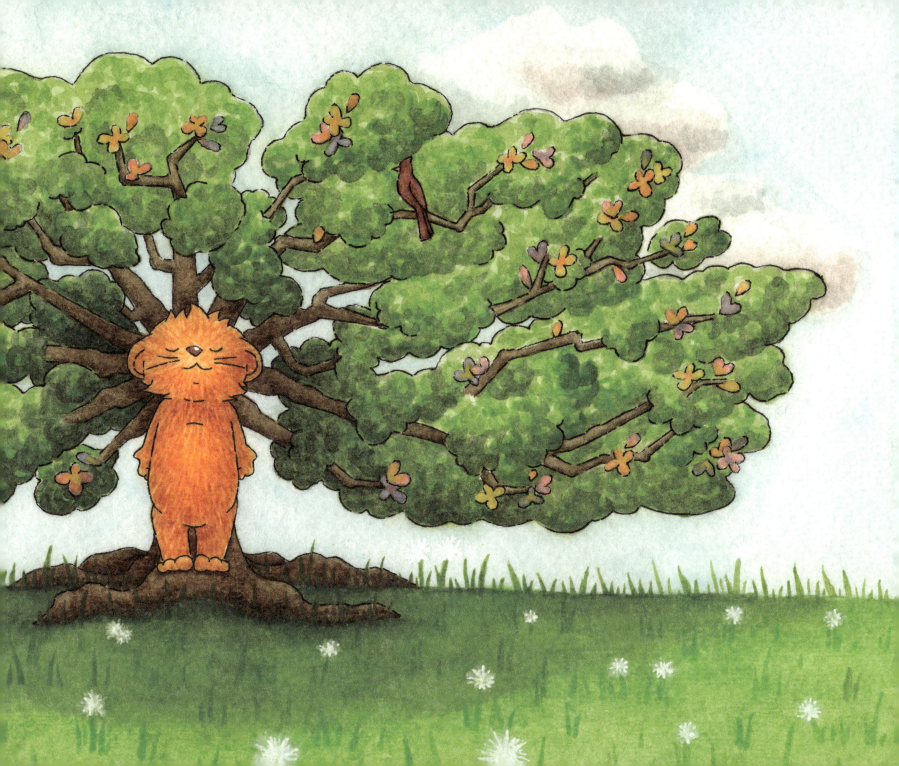

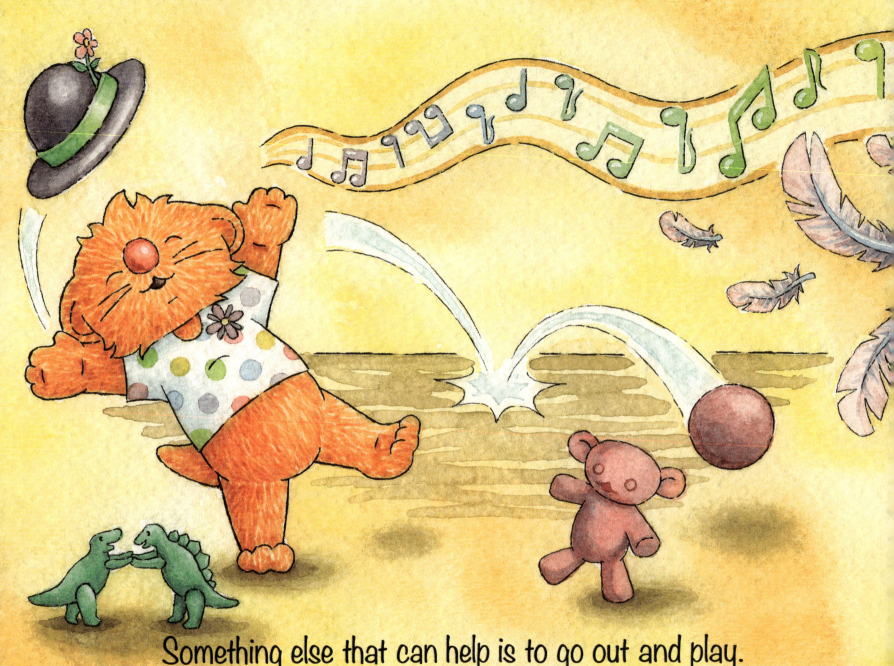

Something else that can help is to go out and play.
It helps me let go of the sad, mad, bad day.

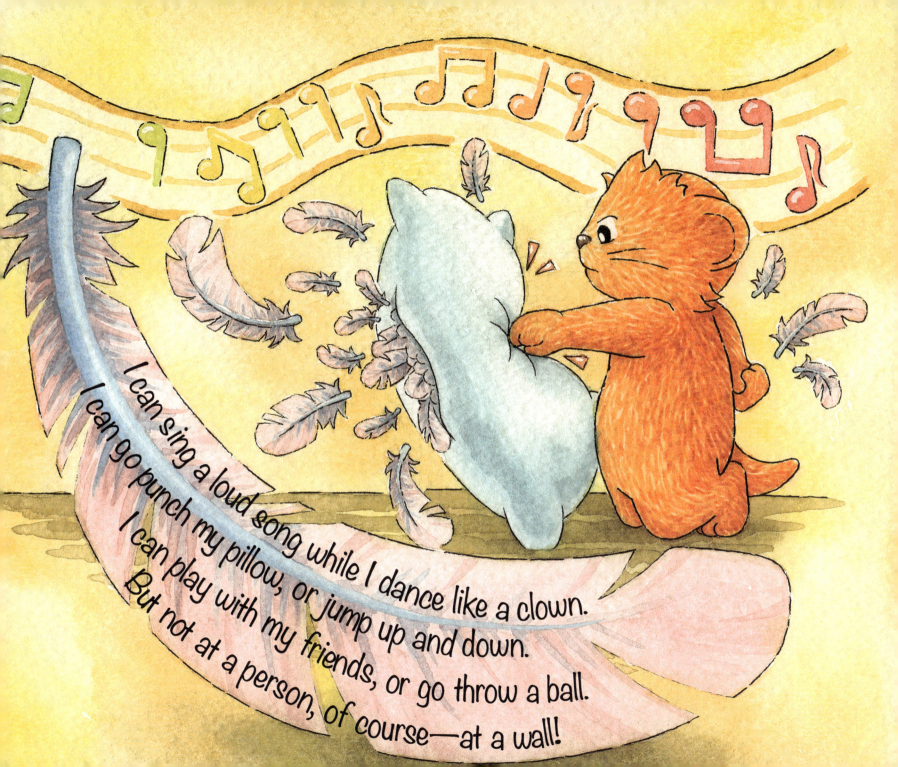

I can sing a loud song while I dance like a clown.
I can go punch my pillow, or jump up and down.
I can play with my friends, or go throw a ball.
But not at a person, of course—at a wall!

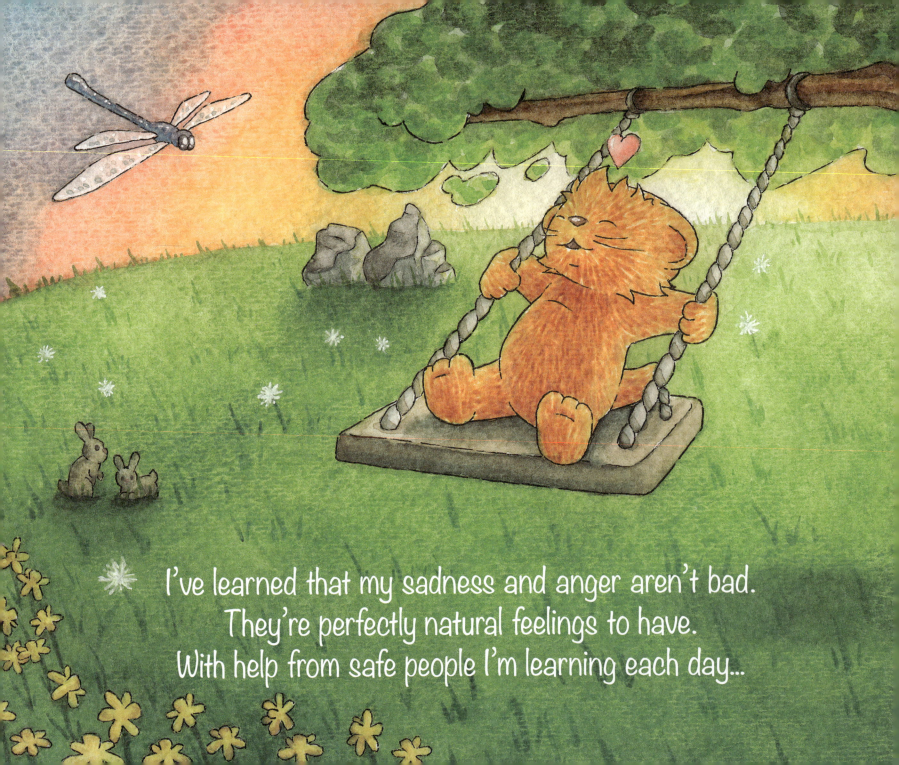

I've learned that my sadness and anger aren't bad.
They're perfectly natural feelings to have.
With help from safe people I'm learning each day...

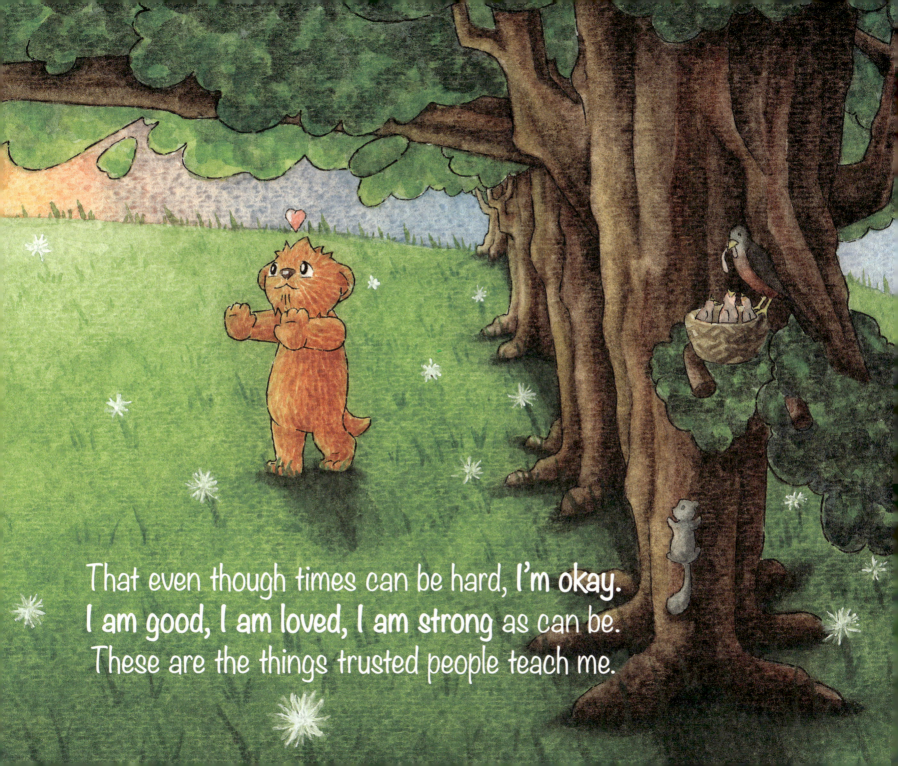

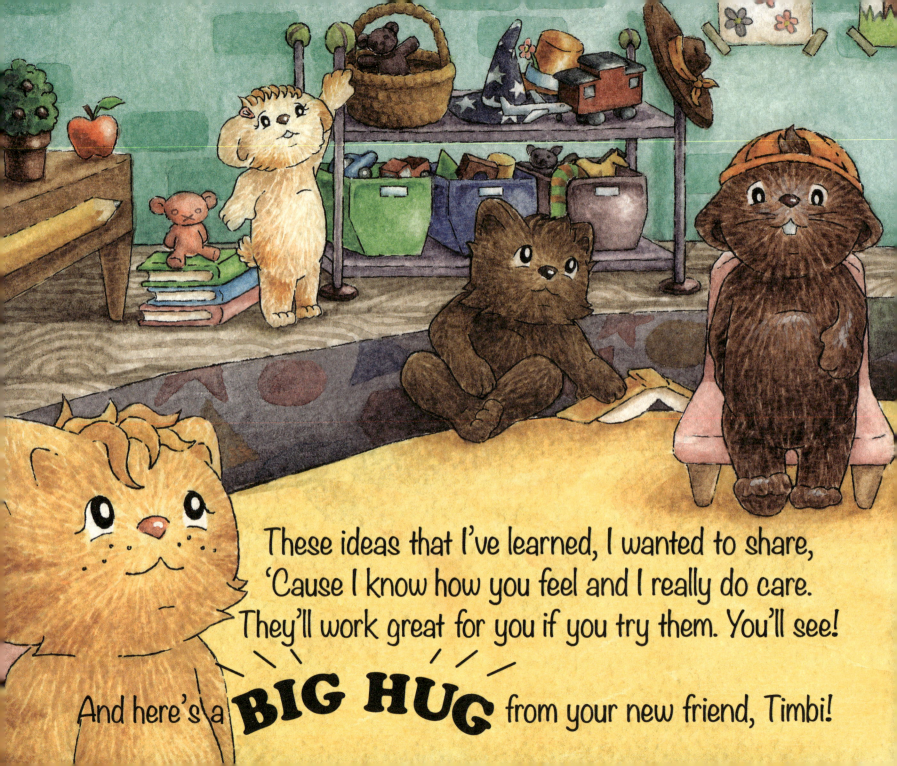

These ideas that I've learned, I wanted to share,
'Cause I know how you feel and I really do care.
They'll work great for you if you try them. You'll see!
And here's a **BIG HUG** from your new friend, Timbi!

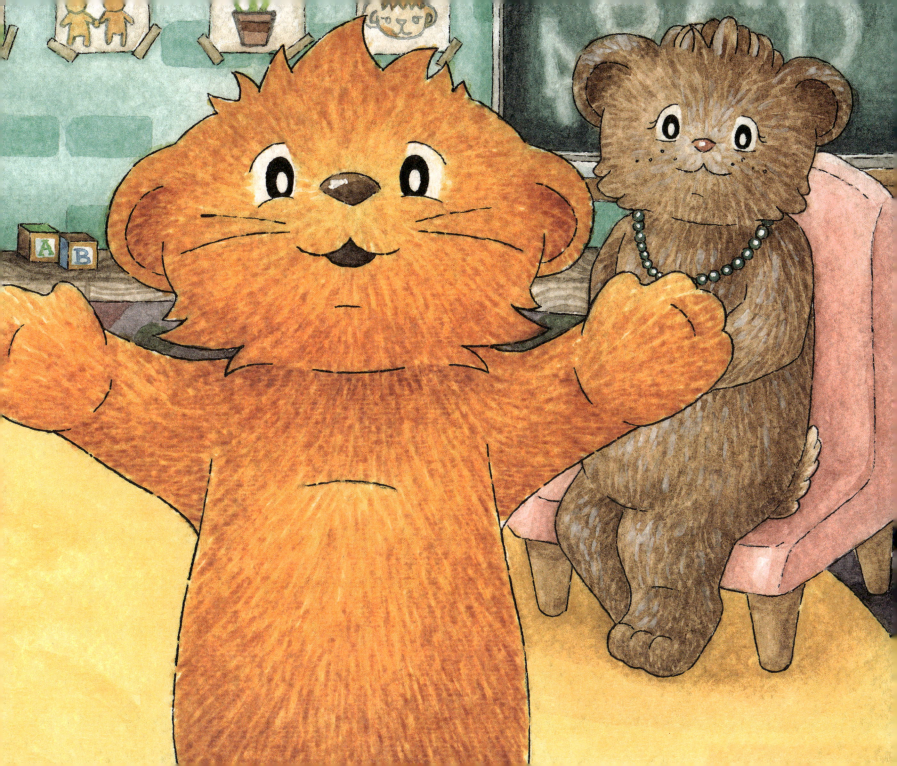

About the Authors

Trish and Janet grew up in New York. Trish now lives in Nashville, Tennessee with her husband, Pat Embry. Trish and Pat have a blended family of four grown children, a daughter-in-law, and three grandchildren. Trish has a master's degree in philosophy and ethics from Vanderbilt University. Janet lives in New York with her husband, John. They have three grown children, and one granddaughter. Janet has a master's degree in mental health counseling.

Trish wrote the first draft of this story, originally titled "My Daddy has a Problem," nearly 30 years ago. Her children, Nick and Sami, had a loving daddy who struggled with addiction his entire life, so Trish knew first-hand the pain and stigma attached to having a loved one who was addicted; she witnessed the impact it had on her children from a very young age. It was important to her that the reality of the disease be addressed directly, and to validate what her children were seeing and feeling.

The current opioid epidemic recalled those difficult years and Trish knew there were still children that needed this book. So, together, word-by-word, Trish and Janet revised and updated Trish's original work, creating and crafting Timbi's character and story. They wanted to ensure *Timbi Talks about Addiction* was an authentic conversation with children who live with the disease of addiction. Janet brought her clinical knowledge as well as her deep appreciation for mindfulness practices, and how those practices can be especially helpful to people living in a chronically stressed environment. They wish to thank their family and friends for their support and encouragement through this labor of love.

About the Illustrator

Mackenzie has been drawing since she was a toddler, but it wasn't until her senior year in high school that she decided she wanted to get serious with her craft and to study art. She graduated with a BFA in New Media and Design at the University of North Carolina at Greensboro, and lives her dream job as a graphic designer and editor. Mackenzie's biggest reward for creating art is seeing the smile on peoples' faces.

About the Designer

Lynette learned from a young age that her Etch A Sketch could take her just about anywhere she wanted to go creatively, and she never outgrew the creative freedom that came with it. Now, with 30 years of award-winning design work, she's still amazed at how much fun she has every day.

Timbi loves sharing ways to calm down and let go of difficult feelings.

YOU CAN TRY THEM, TOO!
YOU CAN...

Talk to safe adults.

Take some deep breaths to feel calmer.

Remember addiction is a disease and not your fault.

Learn to listen when your body says, "Something is not right."

Play outside in nature.

Feel thankful for people, places and things in your life.

Remember to have fun and be silly sometimes.

Play with friends.

Read books.

Hug your Teddy, blanket or other lovey.

Always remember:

You are good. You are loved. You are strong as can be.

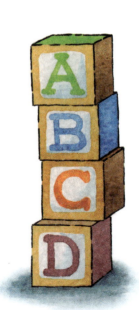

Write a note to Timbi!

Please go to our website and write a note to Timbi and share what works best for you!

Visit: timbitalks.com/note

Timbi would love to hear from you, and might even write you back!

Helpful Information

We know firsthand how hard it can be to find appropriate resources for children who have a parent struggling with addiction. On our website, timbitalks.com, you will find a comprehensive list of websites, books and programs that provide support for children and families. The resources we share have been enormously helpful for us, and we hope they can help guide a child through the difficult challenges addiction creates within the family.

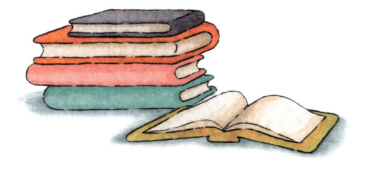
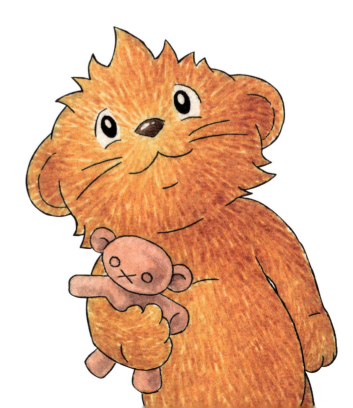

Text and illustration copyright © 2021 by MoonStar Publishing LLC.
www.timbitalks.com

Printed and bound in the United States of America.
10 9 8 7 6 5 4 3 2 1
First Edition

All Rights Reserved. No part of this book may be reproduced
in any form or by any electronic or mechanical means,
including information storage and retrieval systems, without
permission in writing from its publisher, except by a reviewer
who may quote brief passages in the review.

Library of Congress Cataloging-in-Publication data is on file with the publsiher.

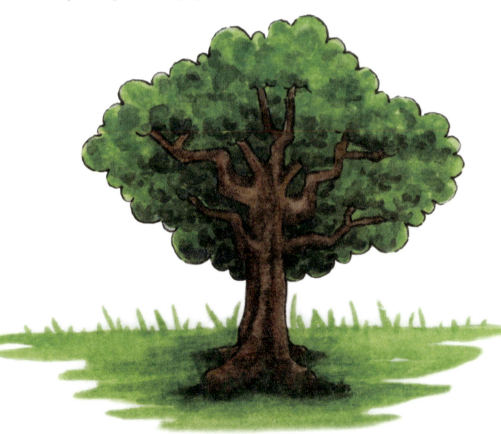